STRENGTH TRAINING

WORKOUTS BIBLE

For Seniors Over 70

Quick And Simple Exercises To Promote Longevity, Enhance Balance, And Boost Mobility

DR. THOMPSON CLARK

Disclaimer

The design of this book is centered on your health and well-being. The exercises, advice, and suggestions are intended to help you on your path to better mobility and relief. Please keep in mind, though, that every person has a unique body, so what suits one may not suit another.

Before beginning any new fitness regimen, I advise speaking with your doctor, particularly if you have any underlying medical issues or concerns. Take it slow and pay attention to your body as you go since your safety comes first.

This book is not a replacement for expert medical advice, diagnosis, or treatment; rather, it is meant to empower and inspire you with strength training strategies. Please contact a licensed healthcare provider if you have any questions or concerns about your health.

I hope this book gives you the inspiration, drive, and doable actions you need to live a more pleasant and active life.

Reader Testimonials...

Here are brief testimonies from readers who found relief and restored mobility with ***"Strength Training Workouts Bible For Seniors Over 70"***

Marjorie, 78, Retired Teacher

I never imagined I could lift weights at my age, but this book altered my perspective completely. I was in my late 70s when I first picked up "Strength Training Workouts Bible For Seniors Over 70" and had no idea where to begin. The exercises are simple to follow and well-suited to my ability. After only a few weeks, my mobility improved, and I was able to get out of my chair without experiencing the normal stiffness in my knees. The progression has been fantastic! I feel stronger, more autonomous, and more confident. This book gave me a new lease on life.

Henry, 72, Retired Mechanic

As a long-time back pain sufferer, I was unconvinced that strength training would work for me. But after reading "The Strength Training Workouts Bible for Seniors Over 70," I gave it a shot. I began with the basic exercises created by my health consultant from the first 20 exercises in this book and was pleasantly surprised at how soon I felt stronger. My back discomfort has subsided, and I feel more active than I have in years. I felt at ease and confident because the book emphasized safe, simple workouts. I'm now enjoying walks and even taking up gardening again, which I never thought I'd do.

Esther, 74, Grandmother of Three

I've tried several workout routines in the past, but none felt right for my age. This book is distinctive. The format is ideal for seniors, gradually increasing effort while focusing on safety and form. I've strengthened my arms and legs, and most significantly, I've restored my confidence. I was able to complete the exercises at my own pace, and the results have been fantastic. I can now walk upstairs without holding onto the railings, and my posture has improved. I wish I'd started sooner.

Each of these readers achieved long-term relief from the book's systematic method, and their stories demonstrate how effective this program can be for individuals of all ages, especially for Seniors over 70.

TABLE OF CONTENTS

ABOUT THE AUTHOR

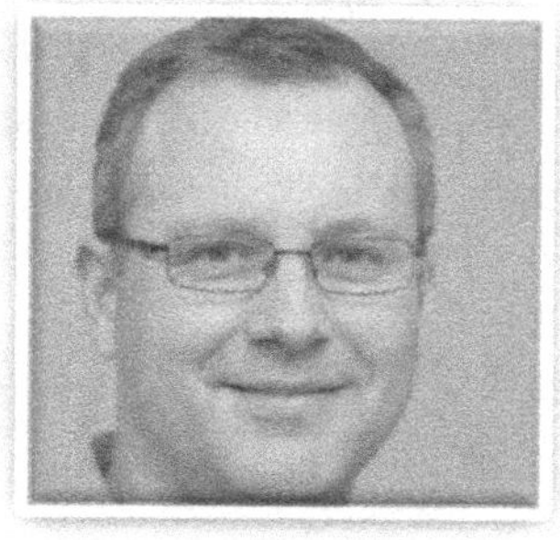

Dr. Thompson Clark is a seasoned physical therapist and geriatric care specialist with over 30 years of experience working to improve the lives of older individuals. Dr. Clark, a specialist in mobility, flexibility, and pain treatment, has established himself as a respected figure in senior health, advocating for non-invasive approaches that assist older people in preserving their freedom. His desire to help seniors stay active and healthy has led him to create simple stretching routines adapted to their specific needs.

Dr. Clark's schooling includes a *Doctorate of Physical Therapy (DPT)* with a focus on geriatric care. Early in his work, he noticed a void in elder healthcare: exercise and mobility were frequently disregarded in favor of medication or surgery. In response, he developed individualized programs to manage chronic pain, flexibility, and posture, allowing individuals of all ages to enjoy pain-free, satisfying lives. His method emphasizes the importance of simple, effective exercises that anyone can undertake, regardless of fitness level.

As an author, Dr. Clark has written extensively about senior health and wellness, making complicated medical concepts simple for his readers. His books and articles highlight the benefits of stretching and movement for older people, providing practical recommendations that seniors can adopt into their everyday routines. His writing has a devoted audience due to his ability to explain health information without compromising depth or accuracy.

In addition to his professional practice and writing, Dr. Clark is a prominent advocate for seniors' mental and emotional well-being. He incorporates mindfulness and relaxation techniques into his stretching sessions, which assist older folks manage stress and anxiety while improving their physical health. His holistic approach emphasizes the link between mind and body, encouraging elders to look after both parts of their well-being.

Dr. Clark is active in his community, providing free workshops and wellness initiatives for seniors, particularly in impoverished regions. His dedication to keeping older individuals active and healthy extends beyond his professional career, as he continues to educate healthcare workers and promote wellness programs that enable seniors to live their best lives.

INTRODUCTION

As I stood outside the gym, a stiff wind blew through the morning air, I noticed Mary, a 73-year-old woman with an engaging smile and a twinkle in her eye, pacing anxiously in front of the facility. She had never set foot in a gym before, let alone considered lifting weights. She had been busy for the majority of her life, raising a family, working, and dealing with the daily grind. But as the years went by, she realized something that many of us do as we get older: aches, pains, stiffness in her joints, and the nagging feeling that things weren't as simple as they used to be.

Mary had heard of strength training for seniors and believed it may benefit her. She had heard stories from friends, newspapers, and even her doctor about the benefits of weight training, such as how it might assist increase mobility, lowering the chance of falls, strengthening bones, and restoring confidence. Nonetheless, a portion of her opposed the idea. *Could she accomplish this? Could lifting weights assist someone like her, who had never been inside a gym? Wasn't strength training only for young people and athletes?*

I approached her, offering a warm handshake and a comforting smile. "Mary," I continued gently, "this marks the beginning of a trip that has the potential to improve your life. Like many others before you, you're about to discover how strength training can make you feel stronger, more capable, and more confident at any age."

Mary's trepidation subsided, and as we entered the gym, I could feel the energy shift. That day was the start of her adventure into strength training. By the end of her first month, she had already seen considerable improvements. Her energy was restored, her back discomfort had subsided, and even ordinary things like carrying groceries were less stressful. But more importantly, Mary had gained something far more valuable: a sense of independence.

This book is intended to take you down the same path. It's intended for people like Mary, those who may be uncertain, who have previously doubted themselves, but who are ready to take the next step toward recovering strength, confidence, and a higher quality of life. This is your chance to repair and succeed.

I've worked with countless seniors who were formerly in Mary's position. They were afraid that their finest years were behind them, that their muscles were too weak or their bodies were too delicate to withstand strength training. Yet, over and again, I've witnessed them overcome their worries. I've seen them grow from nervous novices to empowered individuals who feel more alive than ever before. And I wish the same for you.

Why is Strength Training Important for Seniors?

Muscle mass and strength naturally deteriorate with age. This condition, known as **sarcopenia,** can start as early as our 30s but increases in our 60s and beyond. This loss of muscle mass can cause a range of problems, including decreased mobility, an increased risk of falling, and even trouble with daily tasks like carrying groceries or getting out of a chair. But there's good news: strength training can help reverse this trend. It's not just about developing huge muscles; it's also about retaining the strength required for a healthy, independent lifestyle.

Strength exercise benefits seniors by increasing muscular mass while also improving bone density, joint function, balance, and flexibility. It's about improving your ability to live without limits, whether that's climbing stairs, getting out of a chair without help, or simply carrying a bag of shopping. And, as you'll see in the next chapters, strength training is entirely customizable to your fitness level.

The exercises in this book were created with you in mind. Whether you're a complete novice or have been exercising for years, there's something here to meet you where you are. The journey ahead will be unique to each individual, but the outcomes are universal: increased strength, improved health, and more freedom to enjoy life as you age.

Like Mary, many readers have shared their stories with me throughout the years. Tom, a guy, had suffered from arthritis for decades. His knees were stiff, and walking was sometimes unpleasant. But after a few months of strength training, he was able to take regular walks without discomfort and even resumed gardening, a hobby he had abandoned years before. He told me that not only had his joints improved, but his entire perspective on life had shifted. He no longer felt dependent on his body. Instead, he felt like he had control.

Another reader, Helen, was concerned that strength training would be too strenuous on her heart. She had a history of heart illness and had always avoided strenuous exercise. However, after consulting with her doctor, she realized that strength training could potentially improve her heart health. Helen was able to raise her energy levels, sleep better, and even drop her blood pressure after a few weeks of implementing a consistent, personalized strength training routine.

Stories like this are why I'm so eager to share this book with you. Strength training has transformed the lives of countless seniors, and I believe it can do the same for you. If you want to relieve pain, enhance mobility, or simply feel stronger in your daily life, this book will walk you through the process step by step.

I realize how difficult it can be to take the initial step. It might be stressful to consider starting something new, especially when it requires a little sweat and work. But I promise you that, like Mary, Tom, Helen, and so many others, you are capable of more than you realize. Strength training for seniors focuses on progress rather than perfection. It's about doing your best today and improving tomorrow.

So, I welcome you to embark on this trip with me. Each chapter is a step closer to becoming a stronger, healthier, and more independent version of yourself. As you work through these exercises, keep in mind that every rep, set, and stretch is about more than simply physical strength; it's also about developing a new relationship with yourself. You're regaining your health, confidence, and future.

Let us begin the path to repair and prosper together.

CHAPTER 1: COMPREHENDING SENIOR STRENGTH TRAINING

An Overview Of The Health Effects Of Age-Related Muscle Loss

Our bodies naturally alter as we age, impacting our metabolism, muscles, bones, and general well-being. The gradual loss of muscle mass and strength, medically referred to as sarcopenia, is one of the most noticeable of these alterations. Age-related muscle loss impacts nearly every bodily system, including balance, movement, metabolism, and even mental health.

Sarcopenia is the age-related progressive loss of muscle mass, strength, and function. While muscular atrophy can start in our thirties, sarcopenia typically manifests in those over 60 and speeds up around age 70. The term is Greek, with *sarx* meaning *"flesh"* and *penia* meaning *"loss."* Studies show that adults lose roughly 3-8% of their muscle mass every ten years after the age of 30 and that this rate rises with age.

Reasons for Muscle Loss with Age

1. Decreased Physical Activity: A lack of physical activity, especially strength training and resistance exercise, is one of the main causes of sarcopenia. Although muscle tissue adapts well to use and stress, muscles atrophy and decrease when not utilized regularly.

2. Hormonal Changes: As people age, their levels of growth hormone, estrogen, and testosterone sometimes fluctuate. It is more difficult to build and maintain muscle when these hormone levels decline because they are crucial for preserving muscle mass.

3. Decreased Protein Synthesis: As we get older, our bodies' capacity to produce protein from food and allocate it to muscle tissue appropriately deteriorates. This implies that older people may not successfully build muscle even with a high-protein diet.

4. Chronic Inflammation: Low-level, ongoing inflammation is common in the elderly and has a role in the deterioration of muscles. By progressively weakening muscles, inflammatory diseases like arthritis can hasten this decline.

5. Neurological Changes: As people age, their neuromuscular system may be impacted. This could lead to a decrease in the number of nerve signals that reach their muscles, which

would decrease their function and responsiveness. Muscular strength and coordination are directly impacted by the loss of nerve function and muscle stimulation.

Impacts on Life Quality and Health

The effects of muscle loss on physical, metabolic, and mental health are extensive. The following are some of the primary ways that sarcopenia impacts general health:

1. Decreased Mobility and Balance: One's capacity to move freely and maintain balance is hampered by a loss of muscle strength. The risk of falling and breaking could increase if even basic activities like walking, climbing stairs, or moving out of a seated position become challenging. One of the main causes of injury and diminished independence among the elderly is falls.

2. Increased Risk of Fracture and Bone Loss: Because muscles and bones cooperate, the forces that muscles apply help maintain stable bone density. Bones are not appropriately stressed as muscle mass declines, raising the risk of osteoporosis, bone fractures, and other skeletal conditions.

3. Muscles burn calories even when they are not in motion since they are metabolically active tissues. Weight gain and a higher risk of metabolic diseases like type 2 diabetes are common outcomes of a decrease in muscle mass, which also

causes a decrease in metabolic rate. The body's energy balance can be maintained, and metabolic function can be preserved by maintaining a healthy muscular mass.

4. Decreased Independence and Quality of Life: One's ability to live independently may be diminished by the physical limitations brought on by muscle loss. Simple tasks like cleaning, gardening, and grocery shopping have become challenging or impossible, which has an impact on one's self-esteem and quality of life.

5. Elevated Risk for Chronic Illnesses: Muscle mass affects metabolic health in general. A higher risk of chronic conditions like diabetes, heart disease, high blood pressure, and several types of cancer has been linked to muscle loss. Since muscles retain glucose, their loss can result in insulin resistance, a key risk factor for diabetes and heart disease.

6. A person's mental health may suffer as a result of physical limitations and restricted freedom. Elderly people who lose muscle may also feel helpless, have a higher fear of falling, and have a worse sense of self-worth. Since exercise improves brain health and cognitive function, a decrease in physical activity might worsen depression and cognitive decline.

How to Stop and Handle Age-Related Muscle Loss

The good news is that there are efficient ways to stop or lessen muscle loss, and sarcopenia is not irreversible.

1. Strength Training: One of the best ways to fight sarcopenia is to engage in regular strength training activities including bodyweight exercises, resistance band workouts, and weightlifting. At any age, strength training can help you build muscle and improve your strength, endurance, and muscle mass.

2. Sufficient Protein Consumption: To increase muscle synthesis, older adults require more protein than younger ones. Lean meats, fish, eggs, beans, and lentils are examples of foods high in protein that can support the maintenance of muscle mass. Protein supplements may be helpful for certain people, but they should only be taken under a doctor's supervision.

3. Remaining Active: In addition to strength training, regular exercise like riding, swimming, or walking can help preserve general fitness and muscle function. Additionally, exercise enhances mental health, balance, and cardiovascular health.

4. Resolving Hormonal Imbalance: Speaking with a healthcare professional about their hormone levels may be beneficial for certain individuals. Hormone balance may occasionally

be improved by treatments and lifestyle modifications, but these must be carefully managed.

5. Managing Chronic Conditions: Muscle loss can be avoided by effectively managing long-term health issues like diabetes, heart disease, and arthritis. Maintaining strength and mobility requires treating these issues since they can cause inflammation and inactivity.

6. Calcium and Vitamin D Intake: The health of bones and muscles depends on both calcium and vitamin D. Enough vitamin D from food, supplements, or sunlight can support healthy aging. Vitamin D aids in muscular function and calcium absorption.

As people age, there are significant advantages to taking preventative measures to maintain muscle mass early in life. Strength training can help maintain independence, vitality, and quality of life while preventing muscle loss when combined with a nutritious diet and an active lifestyle. By including strength training, a healthy diet, and regular exercise in their daily routines, seniors can preserve their mobility and good health far into old age.

Although age-related muscle loss is common, it is also very manageable. Overall health can be greatly improved by understanding the significance of muscular health, identifying the causes of sarcopenia, and putting prevention strategies into practice. Muscle preservation is crucial for adults over 70 to keep their independence, avoid chronic illnesses, and live better lives in addition to being physically active. Aging adults can flourish and maintain an active lifestyle into their older years by preventing the impacts of muscle loss with awareness and consistent effort.

Strength Training's Advantages For Seniors

With its many advantages that enhance independence, quality of life, and overall health, strength training is becoming recognized as a useful technique for adults over 70. Research and personal experience demonstrate that seniors can significantly benefit from adding resistance exercises to their regimens, even though strength training has historically been linked to younger populations or sports. Let's examine a few of the main advantages of strength training for seniors.

1. Keeping strength and preventing muscle loss

The natural aging-related loss of muscle mass is known as sarcopenia. Around age 30, muscle mass starts to decline at a rate of 3-5% per ten years, which quickens beyond age 60. Strength, balance, and mobility may be compromised by this gradual muscle degradation, raising the possibility of falls and injuries. One of the best ways for seniors to stop or even reverse muscle loss is through strength training. This will help them maintain their muscle mass and functional strength, which are necessary for everyday tasks like carrying groceries, getting out of a chair, and walking on their own.

By focusing on particular muscle regions, strength training exercises enhance tone and encourage the creation of new muscle fibers. Elderly people can preserve and even regain muscle mass with low-impact exercises using resistance bands or small weights. Elderly people can move more confidently since this strength preservation creates the foundation for greater physical resilience and independence.

2. Reduced risk of osteoporosis and increased bone density

People's bones deteriorate with age and are more prone to breaking. The condition known as osteoporosis, which is characterized by weak and brittle bones, is common among older people, especially women. Strength training is a wonderful way to strengthen bones because it applies controlled stress to the skeleton, which activates bone-forming cells. Over time, this "stress" causes the body to produce more calcium deposits in the bones, which increases bone density.

Bone strengthening reduces the risk of fractures, which is particularly important for elderly people because bone fractures can cause long recovery periods and limited mobility. Seniors who engage in regular resistance training can maintain stronger, healthier bones and reduce their risk of osteoporosis-related fractures, especially those that affect the hips, spine, and wrists.

3. Better pain management and joint health

Seniors frequently experience joint pain and stiffness, and many have conditions like arthritis. By strengthening the muscles surrounding the joints, strength training helps to control and lessen joint pain by increasing support and easing the load on the troublesome areas. Strong muscles help to release pressure from the joints, making movement more comfortable and painless. Exercises designed specifically for seniors are often gentle and low-impact, which makes them appropriate for people with arthritis or other joint-related conditions.

Strength exercise can also help lower inflammation in the body. Joint and muscle pain is frequently made worse by chronic inflammation, and it has been discovered that regular exercise—particularly resistance training—reduces inflammation markers. Seniors who follow a consistent routine may find that their joints become less painful and tight, enabling them to move more easily.

4. Better balance and a decreased chance of falling

Seniors are frequently injured and admitted to hospitals due to falls, which frequently result in a decline in their independence and standard of living. Because of muscle weakness and a decline in proprioception—the body's sense of location and movement—balance and coordination typically degrade with age. Balance and stability are essential for preventing falls, and they can be enhanced with strength training exercises that prioritize leg strength, core stability, and functional motions.

Lower body activities that strengthen the legs and core, like sitting leg lifts, toe taps, and resistance band exercises, improve balance. Seniors who strengthen their lower body and core muscles have better coordination and greater control over their motions. Seniors may feel more secure when walking and climbing stairs thanks to their increased stability and balance, which could reduce their risk of falling.

5. Improved heart health

Although strength training is frequently linked to muscular growth, it also has positive effects on heart health. Resistance training increases circulation, which supports heart and blood vessel health. Additionally, strength training lowers blood pressure, raises cholesterol, and facilitates better blood flow. Strength training can be a crucial component of maintaining cardiovascular health for seniors who are already at risk for heart disease.

Particularly useful for regulating blood sugar levels, strength training can aid in the management or prevention of type 2 diabetes. During resistance training, glucose is used as an energy source when muscles contract, lowering blood sugar and increasing insulin sensitivity. Seniors with diabetes or at risk for the disease might maintain healthy blood sugar levels by engaging in strength training.

6. Benefits to mental health and cognitive function

Strength training has major psychological effects in addition to physical ones. Exercise, such as resistance training, promotes the release of endorphins, which are feel-good and stress-relieving chemicals. Frequent exercise can help reduce the symptoms of anxiety and depression that are frequent in older adults, particularly in those who feel alone or have aging-related problems.

Moreover, cognitive functioning can be improved through muscle training. Research indicates that resistance training increases blood flow to the brain and triggers the synthesis of neurotrophic chemicals, which support cognitive function and neuronal health. Frequent exercise may help prevent dementia and has been linked to slower cognitive decline. Seniors over 70 who engage in strength training can enhance their mood, focus, and mental clarity in addition to their physical resilience.

7. Increased flexibility and mobility

Strength training increases range of motion, flexibility, muscle tone, and stability. Seniors can preserve or improve their mobility by engaging in strength workouts that often incorporate joint movement over a range of motions. Elderly people need flexibility to avoid stiffness and to be able to perform daily tasks with ease.

Exercises that keep muscles stretched and joints supple include leg lifts, lunges, and resistance band stretches. Seniors may move with confidence and freedom because it combines strength and flexibility, which encourages a more active lifestyle. Elderly people with increased mobility can also engage in family activities, travel, and hobbies that would otherwise be challenging.

8. Enhanced vitality and quality of sleep

Additionally, strength training helps improve the quality of sleep, which is commonly problematic for elderly people. The body's internal clock is regulated by physical activity, which makes it easier to fall asleep and stay asleep through the night. Additionally, it helps improve sleep by lessening the symptoms of sleep disorders including anxiety and sleep apnea, which can both interfere with sleep cycles. Better sleep promotes an active and involved lifestyle by increasing alertness and energy during the day.

Strength training also increases the effectiveness of the muscular and cardiovascular systems, which raises energy levels. Elderly people who have stronger muscles and a healthy circulatory system will feel more energized and less exhausted on a regular basis.

9. Encourage social interaction

Strength training can support greater community and social interaction, all of which are critical for mental health and overall enjoyment. Many senior citizens participate in local community centers or group fitness programs, which provide chances for support and social connection.

These social connections can aid in the fight against isolation and loneliness, which are common among the elderly. Developing connections with individuals who share your fitness objectives boosts accountability and drive, which makes working out more enjoyable. Moreover, the companionship fostered in group settings enhances emotional health and a feeling of inclusion, so elevating the general quality of life.

10. Generating a feeling of achievement

Strength training increases your self-confidence and provides you with a sense of satisfaction when you reach your fitness goals. These successes, whether they include learning a new skill, increasing repetitions, or lifting heavier weights, increase self-esteem and cultivate a can-do attitude.

Seniors who experience this sense of accomplishment may be inspired to take on new challenges, engage in hobbies, or get involved in community activities. Strength training helps seniors enjoy life with passion and joy by boosting their confidence, which in turn improves resilience and encourages a proactive attitude to aging.

11. Establishing a structure and routine

Weekly strength training gives you a sense of purpose and organization, which is particularly helpful when you're retired or have less time to exercise. Seniors who stick to a regular training schedule become more disciplined and are inspired to put their health and well-being first.

Additionally, a structured exercise program can improve sleep patterns, which raises happiness and vitality levels all around. Recuperation, cognitive function, and emotional regulation all depend on getting enough good sleep, which helps people live longer and in better health.

People over 70 can benefit from strength training in many ways, including better mental and physical health. By maintaining muscle mass, boosting bone density, enhancing mobility, and supporting cardiovascular health, strength training enables older adults to lead more active and fulfilling lives. A senior's program should include strength training for several reasons, such as improved mental health, improved balance, and less pain. Strength training is a safe and effective way for seniors to stay healthy and active far into old age, regardless of their degree of experience.

Dispelling Myths And Misunderstandings About Strength Training For Senior Citizens

As we age, our bodies undergo changes that might affect our strength, balance, and overall level of fitness. For many elders, strength training on a regular basis enhances their independence, health, and quality of life. Nevertheless, despite the advantages, many older people are discouraged from participating in strength training due to persistent beliefs and misconceptions. In order to help elders view strength training as a secure and efficient means of preserving their health and vitality, it is imperative that these misconceptions be addressed.

Myth 1: Seniors should avoid strength training

Due to concerns about potential harm, one of the most widespread myths is that strength training is risky for senior citizens. Proper strength training is not only safe but also useful, even if seniors may be more susceptible to certain illnesses. Research has repeatedly demonstrated that older adults who strength exercise experience fewer injuries than those who do not.

Good technique and a tailored training program that considers each person's unique abilities, limitations, and health concerns are the first steps toward safety. Working with a qualified trainer who specializes in instructing senior citizens might help them avoid overtraining and develop proper form. Additionally, adaptation is possible without putting undue strain on the body by beginning with small weights or resistance bands and progressively increasing intensity.

Myth 2: Bulky muscles are the result of strength training

Another common misconception is that strength training results in large muscles, which many elderly people would rather not have. Women are particularly prone to this misunderstanding because they fear that strength training may make them seem too macho or strong.

It's important to keep in mind that building significant muscle growth requires certain exercise regimens, including using larger weights for fewer repetitions, which are usually coupled with exacting dietary techniques. With conventional strength training programs, the majority of seniors will not gain a large frame. Rather than adding weight, strength training enhances functional mobility, boosts metabolism, builds lean muscle mass, and improves overall strength.

Myth 3: Heavy weights should not be used by elderly people

Many seniors mistakenly believe that anything larger could injure them, thus they should only use small weights. The notion that older people should completely avoid using heavier weights is untrue, even though it is crucial to begin with smaller ones.

Studies have shown that progressive resistance training, which entails progressively increasing weight or resistance as strength increases, is crucial for the development of muscle and bone density. For older people, lifting heavier weights under supervision and in a safe environment can be quite helpful. It helps prevent bone density loss (osteoporosis) and age-related muscle loss (sarcopenia) while also boosting muscle strength. The objective is to use heavier weights carefully and under close supervision, making sure that the workouts are suitable for the person's health and fitness level.

Myth 4: Only young people should engage in strength training.

Strength training, according to many older individuals, is mostly for young, athletic people. Social representations of fitness, which rarely show elderly individuals doing strength training, maybe the source of this misconception.

Strength training helps people of all ages, but especially older adults. It enhances balance, coordination, and overall functional capacity in day-to-day activities in addition to maintaining muscular mass and strength. By increasing mobility and reducing the risk of falls, strength training can help seniors stay active and independent.

Myth 5: Cardio is sufficient to maintain fitness

Some elderly people believe that strength training is superfluous and that aerobic exercises like swimming or walking are sufficient to keep them in shape. Cardiovascular exercise does not increase bone density or muscle strength, but it is beneficial for heart health and endurance.

A comprehensive approach to health requires strength training. Strength training improves muscular tone, boosts metabolism, and encourages good body mechanics, all of which enhance cardiovascular exercise. The greatest health results can be obtained with a well-rounded program that includes both strength and aerobic exercise, enhancing lifespan and quality of life.

Myth 6: Strength training requires a gym membership

The idea of going to a gym may frighten many elderly people because they believe that strength training necessitates having access to certain equipment. However, strength training may be readily adapted to a number of environments, including the comfort of one's own home.

Dumbbells, resistance bands, and even bodyweight exercises can be used for strength training without the need for pricey gym equipment. Seniors can incorporate strength training into their daily routines without the stress of a gym setting by performing easy exercises like chair squats, wall push-ups, and seated leg lifts at home. Furthermore, community facilities and outdoor areas usually offer group classes that foster social skills and responsibility.

Myth 7: Individuals with chronic conditions should not engage in strength training

A common misconception among seniors with long-term medical concerns is that strength training is unaffordable. Health issues may worsen as a result of sedentary behavior brought on by this misconception. Several chronic illnesses, such as diabetes, heart disease, and arthritis, can be treated with strength training.

Strength training can enhance joint function, cardiovascular health, and weight control when paired with a targeted exercise program and appropriate medical guidance. Before starting any new exercise program, seniors should speak with their healthcare provider to make sure it fits their needs. After that, a knowledgeable fitness expert may create a program that safely includes strength training while accounting for any limitations.

Myth 8: To see results, you need to train daily

The idea that seniors need to do strength training daily in order to see improvements is another common fallacy. This misconception may lead to exhaustion and discourage elderly people from starting or maintaining an exercise regimen.

The majority of experts advise seniors to engage in strength training two to three times a week. This frequency offers the right amount of recovery time, which is necessary for both muscle growth and regeneration. Although strength training may not yield immediate benefits, regular application over time results in significant improvements in strength, mobility, and general health.

In order to encourage older people to lead healthier and more active lives, it is essential to dispel myths and misconceptions about strength training. Strength training offers several benefits, from improved bone density and muscle strength to improved balance and quality of life.

We can help seniors achieve their maximum potential for longevity, independence, and health by dispelling these beliefs and promoting safe, supervised strength exercises. It becomes clear that age is only a number as we stress the value of strength training and that being active is beneficial and attainable at any age.

CHAPTER 2: GETTING READY FOR YOUR STRENGTH TRAINING ADVENTURE

Using Self-Assessment Tools Or Advice To Determine Your Level Of Fitness

A crucial first step in any fitness program is determining your current level of fitness, particularly for seniors beginning a strength training program. Understanding your current level of strength, flexibility, endurance, and general health can help you create a safe and effective exercise program that meets your specific needs and objectives. This lesson will cover useful self-assessment techniques and consultation techniques to help you determine your level of fitness.

Before starting any fitness program, especially for seniors, it's important to assess your present level of fitness. This will help you stay motivated, prevent injuries, and make your exercises more successful. Evaluations help in the following ways:

1. To determine your strengths and shortcomings: By understanding your areas of strength and improvement, you may design a training program that is more targeted and successful.

2. To establish reasonable objectives: Fitness evaluations provide a standard by which to gauge progress. You may be able to maintain your motivation and focus by setting reasonable goals that are based on where you are starting.

3. To monitor your progress: Frequent evaluations will help you see your progress and motivate you to continue pursuing your fitness goals.

Self-Evaluations to Determine Fitness Levels

Self-assessments, which don't require specialized equipment or expert guidance, can be a useful way to examine your fitness. Consider the following helpful self-checks:

1. Evaluation of Strengths

❖ Try performing push-ups or squats. Determine the number of tasks you can finish in a minute. Muscle strength and endurance are evaluated by this simple test.

❖ You can perform chest presses and seated rows using resistance bands. Find the resistance level that you can tolerate with ease and still retain proper form.

2. Evaluation of Flexibility

❖ Sit on the floor with your legs straight in front of you to perform the sit-and-reach test. Go forward and touch your toes. Find out how far you can go. This test assesses lower back and hamstring flexibility.

❖ To test your shoulder flexibility, stand up and extend one arm behind your back and one over your shoulder. Calculate how far apart your hands are. This aids in evaluating shoulder suppleness.

3. Evaluation of Balance

❖ Without help, stand for as long as you can on one leg. Note the time in your diary. As your balance improves, progressively extend the time spent on each leg from the first 10 seconds.

❖ Put one foot in front of the other and keep it there to do a tandem stand. You're doing great if you can maintain this posture for ten seconds without slipping!

4. Evaluation of Cardiovascular Endurance

❖ Keep track of how long it takes you to walk a mile at a comfortable pace. You've built up a respectable foundation of cardiovascular endurance if you can complete it in 20 minutes.

❖ Find a sturdy platform or step. After three minutes of stepping up and down, check your heart rate. High cardiovascular fitness is demonstrated by a quick recovery.

5. Evaluation of Core Strengths

❖ For as long as you can, keep your forearms and toes in a plank posture. This test assesses stability and core strength.

❖ Raise your legs off the floor while seated in a chair. Find out how long you can stay in this role. This displays stability and core strength.

Advice for Professional Assessment Consultation

Self-assessments are helpful, but seeing a fitness expert or medical professional can enhance your evaluation and provide you with a more comprehensive view of your current level of fitness. The following rules can help ensure that consultations are successful:

1. Seek certified exercise physiologists, physical therapists, or fitness trainers who have worked with senior citizens. Their expertise allows them to provide customized evaluations and suggestions.

2. Learn about your medical history, current prescriptions, and any previous surgeries or injuries before speaking with a professional. The expert will be able to modify their evaluation to meet your unique needs with this information.

3. Don't be scared to ask questions about the evaluation procedure, what to anticipate, and how your training plan will be developed using the data. You will feel more empowered and maintain your enthusiasm in your fitness journey if you comprehend the rationale behind each test.

4. Talk about your fitness objectives, such as increasing your strength, stamina, or flexibility. Professionals can develop a program that aligns with their objectives when there is clear communication between them.

5. To ascertain your ability to complete daily chores, a specialist might perform functional exams. These assessments help you pinpoint particular training program areas to concentrate on.

6. Schedule frequent consultations with your fitness expert to assess your development and modify your training regimen as necessary. Regular evaluations can keep you accountable and motivated.

Including Evaluations in Your Fitness Path

You must incorporate the results of your self-assessment or consultation into your strength training program after determining your current level of fitness. Here's how to accomplish this:

1. Using the data acquired, create a program that takes into account both your advantages and disadvantages. While maintaining your strengths, focus on areas that need work.

2. Using the findings of your evaluation, establish SMART goals: specific, measurable, achievable, relevant, and time-bound. For instance, aim to perform five more bodyweight squats in four weeks.

3. Every few months, reevaluate your level of fitness to track your progress. Celebrate your successes and adjust your workouts and goals as necessary.

4. Be prepared to alter your training schedule as you advance. Pay attention to your body, and seek professional advice on how to adjust if you are feeling tired or uncomfortable.

5. You may maintain consistency in your workouts by doing regular evaluations. Making improvements can boost your self-esteem and motivate you to maintain your fitness objectives.

For seniors beginning a strength training program, determining your level of fitness through self-tests and consultations is a crucial first step. You can modify your workouts to be safe, efficient, and in line with your fitness objectives by being aware of your current ability level. Knowing where you stand will help you make better decisions regarding your fitness and health objectives, regardless of whether you decide to evaluate yourself or seek professional advice. Accept this process and keep in mind that you are getting closer to being a healthier, better version of yourself with every step you take.

The Equipment Needed For Senior Strength Training Exercises

Strength training helps reverse age-related muscle loss, boosts bone density, improves mobility, and fosters independence, making it a crucial component of senior health and fitness, especially for those over 70. However, it is essential to comprehend the various kinds of equipment that are available, their benefits, and how to use them safely and effectively before starting a strength training program. Popular senior-friendly strength training tools like dumbbells, resistance bands, bodyweight exercises, and safety mats will be covered in this equipment overview.

1. Dumbbells

Dumbbells are small, lightweight weights that come in a variety of sizes, from one to fifty pounds. Because of their great versatility, they can be used for a variety of exercises that focus on different muscle areas. Seniors should start with lighter weights (1 to 5 pounds) and gradually raise them as their strength and self-assurance improve.

Dumbbell exercises include weighted squats, shoulder presses, tricep extensions, and bicep curls. Use proper form to prevent harm. Seniors should exercise carefully, focusing on their posture and grip to prevent back or wrist discomfort.

2. Resistance Bands

Resistance bands are elastic bands that, when stretched, provide varying amounts of resistance. They are perfect for seniors who don't have much room for exercise equipment because they are lightweight and portable. The thickness of resistance bands varies, indicating the amount of resistance they offer.

Exercises like seated rows, chest presses, and leg extensions can all be performed using resistance bands. For added support, they can be looped around a chair or fastened to a sturdy object. Seniors should make sure the band is securely fastened before beginning any exercises to prevent it from snapping back and causing injury. It's also crucial to keep an eye on the bands' condition and swap them out if they show signs of wear or damage.

3. Exercises using only body weight

Body weight exercises provide resistance by using the weight of the individual. These exercises are very beneficial for improving flexibility, strength, and balance. Common bodyweight exercises include planks, push-ups, lunges, and squats.

For seniors, chair squats, wall push-ups, and seated leg lifts are excellent beginning exercises. You can modify these exercises to fit different levels of fitness. Keeping the right form is essential to preventing injury. To progressively build strength, seniors should start with easier variations, like wall push-ups rather than regular push-ups.

4. Mats for safety

Safety mats reduce the chance of damage during activities by offering a cushioned surface that can absorb impact. For the elderly, who may be more susceptible to falls and accidents, they are especially important.

Safety mats can be set up in designated training spaces, particularly for stretches and floor exercises. The mat should be placed on a level surface to prevent slipping. Regularly check the mat for wear and tear and replace it as necessary to guarantee safety.

5. Chairs and Equipment for Stability

Many workouts benefit from the support and stability that a sturdy chair provides. Exercises like chair squats and sitting leg lifts can be performed in a chair while seated or while balanced. Additional stability tools, like stability balls or balance cushions, can also aid in enhancing stability and core strength.

Senior exercises include leg lifts, seated arm curls, and chair-assisted modified sit-to-stand exercises. Balance cushions can be used for stability training, while stability balls can be used for seated core exercises. Steer clear of chairs that could slide or topple over and make sure they are sturdy and secure. Make sure the stability balls are in good condition and sufficiently inflated before using them.

6. Other Equipment Choices

Although the aforementioned equipment offers a solid foundation for strength training, seniors may also want to take into account the following choices, depending on their particular requirements and objectives:

- ❖ Weighted Vests: Bodyweight exercises can be made more challenging by wearing a weighted vest, which adds resistance. Elderly people should start with lighter weights, nevertheless, to avoid needless effort.

- ❖ Foam Rollers: Foam rollers can increase the flexibility and healing of muscles. Following exercise, they might improve mobility and lessen discomfort.

- ❖ Yoga Blocks: By providing support and stability, yoga blocks can aid with a variety of stretches and poses when incorporating flexibility and balance training.

In conclusion, seniors over 70 need to have the right strength training equipment. By learning about the advantages and how to utilize dumbbells, resistance bands, bodyweight exercises, safety mats, and other equipment, seniors can enhance their strength, flexibility, and general quality of life. The exercise experience is improved and elders are encouraged to view strength training as a crucial component of their wellness journey by creating a well-organized and easily accessible workout space. With consistent strength training that prioritizes safety and gradual growth, seniors can restore their strength, independence, and vitality.

The Significance Of Setting Up A Safe, Easily Accessible Exercise Space At Home

For anyone who wishes to maintain or improve their physical fitness, especially seniors, having a safe and convenient place to work out at home is essential. In addition to making working out more enjoyable, a suitable environment also reduces the risk of injury and promotes dedication to a fitness regimen. Here, we examine the many facets and advantages of offering senior citizens a safe, easily accessible training facility.

1. Safety factors

Safety is the main justification for designing a unique training environment. Our risk of injury rises with age, and the setting in which we exercise significantly affects that risk. Untidy or cluttered areas can lead to tripping, falls, and other mishaps. These are some crucial safety considerations.

- ❖ Clear Pathways: Ensure that obstacles such as rugs, furniture, and ornaments are removed from the exercise space. When exercising, a path that is unobstructed and clear encourages safe movement and reduces the risk of falling.

- ❖ Non-Slip Surfaces: If at all possible, equip the exercise space with non-slip flooring or mats. This is particularly important for elderly people who might have trouble staying balanced. You can maintain your balance throughout a variety of stretches and workouts by using non-slip surfaces.

❖ Sufficient Lighting: Any training space must have adequate lighting. To prevent accidents brought on by poor visibility, make sure the area is well-lit. To enhance mood and focus throughout different types of exercises, think about using adjustable lighting.

❖ Equipment that is easily accessible should not require awkward reaching or straining. To prevent damaging bending or stretching, keep any weights, resistance bands, or other items within arm's reach.

2. Accessibility

Designing an exercise area that is accessible is essential, especially for senior citizens. When a place is conveniently accessible, people are more likely to use it. Here's how to make things more accessible:

❖ Location: Pick a conveniently located exercise area, ideally on the home's main floor. Stair-accessible basements and attics should be avoided since they might be frightening and deter regular use.

❖ Flexible Layout: Arrange the space to support a range of exercises and motions. It is appropriate for a range of fitness levels due to its customizable layout, which permits both standing and sitting activities.

❖ Supportive Furniture: Set up benches or seats that are comfortable to relax on during sitting workouts or in between exercises. Elderly people may become more involved as a result of knowing they may rest peacefully if needed.

❖ Variety of Equipment: Ensure that the training space has a range of equipment suitable for various skill levels and fitness levels. This might be a yoga mat, stability balls, resistance bands, or even small dumbbells. Seniors can experiment with their training regimens and find what suits them best when they have a variety of possibilities.

3. Psychological benefits

A gym space that is attractive and well-maintained can have a big psychological impact. People are more likely to be motivated and excited to work out when the environment is appealing. Here are a few methods for enhancing the psychological elements:

❖ Personalize the exercise space with plants, motivational sayings, or pictures. These elements can foster a welcoming atmosphere that promotes a positive outlook during training.

❖ Dedicated Space: You may psychologically isolate your workout time from other activities by having a separate training room. This can create a pattern and tell the brain that it's time to put fitness and health first.

❖ Comfortable Temperature: Ensure that the room is maintained at a temperature that is comfortable. Seniors may be discouraged from exercising if it is too hot or too chilly. To create a comfortable atmosphere, think about employing heaters or fans.

❖ Entertainment and music: Some people believe that watching background videos or listening to music improves their workouts. To improve the space's appeal, think about installing a sound system or a tablet that can stream music playlists or exercise DVDs.

4. Promoting consistency

Encouraging consistency in exercise routines also requires designing a training area that is both accessible and safe. A friendly atmosphere can encourage regular workouts, and consistency is key to achieving fitness goals:

❖ Routine Establishment: People can establish a regular exercise routine if they have a specific location. By forming a habit, this regularity makes it simpler to include exercise into your daily schedule.

❖ Decreased Barriers: It is simpler to start an exercise session when everything is prepared and ready to go. Seniors who have a well-organized room are more likely to stick to their fitness regimens and overcome the obstacles that prevent them from working out.

❖ Progress Monitoring: It's simple to monitor your progress when your workstation is well-organized. Seeing progress can boost motivation and encourage consistent effort, whether it's recorded in a notebook or on a chart displayed in the workout area.

5. Social Interaction

Social connection may enhance the whole workout experience for many seniors. There may be more advantages to setting up a space that works for group training:

❖ Think about inviting family members or friends to work out with you. Exercise becomes more enjoyable and less lonely when a shared gym space encourages social contact.

❖ Workshops for groups: If space permits, think about setting up workshops for small groups or asking instructors to conduct sessions. Participants may develop a sense of accountability and community as a result.

❖ Virtual Engagement: Virtual exercises are popular in today's digital world. Make sure the setting is appropriate for video conferences or online courses with loved ones, enabling social interaction even when people are far away.

Seniors who wish to increase their level of fitness and general well-being must set up a safe and convenient home gym. By emphasizing accessibility, and safety, and creating a motivating atmosphere, people can develop a positive relationship with exercise. In addition to lowering the risk of injury, this particular setting encourages regularity and social interaction, which leads to a healthier, more active way of living. The quality of life, confidence, and health of older adults can all be improved by devoting time and energy to designing a first-rate training space.

CHAPTER 3: SAFETY FIRST: ADVICE AND METHODS

Suitable Warm-Up Techniques To Get Joints And Muscles Ready

Any fitness program must include a decent warm-up, but it's especially important for seniors who do strength training. Our flexibility and mobility may be compromised as we age due to changes in our muscles and joints. Warming up is therefore not only beneficial but also essential for preventing injuries and enhancing performance.

The Importance of Warming Up

1. Improves Blood Flow: Warming up causes your heart rate to gradually increase, which enhances blood flow to your muscles. The oxygen and nutrients needed for muscle function are supplied by this increased blood flow, readying the muscles for more demanding activity.

2. Increases Flexibility: Warm-ups aid in making muscles and connective tissues more flexible. By enabling a greater range of motion during exercise, this improved flexibility reduces the risk of sprains and strains.

3. Mental Preparation: You can also psychologically get ready for your workout with a good warm-up. It acts as a break between everyday tasks and exercise, enabling you to focus on your fitness goals and the workouts you plan to perform.

4. Lowers the Risk of Injury: The potential of warm-up activities to lower the risk of injury is one of their most significant benefits. You can lower your chance of injury by progressively increasing the intensity of your workout to give your body time to adjust to the physical demands of the activity.

5. Enhances Performance: Warm-ups done correctly can improve performance in general. You may be able to lift heavier weights or perform exercises with better form when your muscles are properly developed, which could lead to more effective workouts.

Elements of a Successful Warm-Up Program

Active stretching and a general warm-up are often the two main parts of a warm-up routine.

1. General Warm-Up: To increase your heart rate and warm your body, do rhythmic, low-intensity movements. The goal is to increase your heart rate gradually while increasing blood flow.

2. Dynamic Stretching: This technique entails moving certain body parts through their full range of motion once you've warmed up. It facilitates the better preparation of your joints and muscles for the exercises you will be performing.

Example Senior Warm-Up Exercise

These thorough warm-up activities are ideal for seniors and may be finished in 10-15 minutes:

1. Marching or Walking in Place (5 minutes): Start by marching in place or taking a stroll around the room. Focus on naturally swinging your arms and lifting your legs a little.

2. Arm Circles: Hold your arms out to the side while standing or sitting for one minute. After 30 seconds of drawing small circles, switch to the opposite direction for another 30 seconds.

3. Leg Swings (2 minutes): Swing one leg back and forth for 10 to 15 repetitions, then switch legs while holding onto a sturdy surface for support.

4. Body Twists (1 minute): Allow your arms to follow as you gently twist your body from side to side while keeping your feet shoulder-width apart. Take a minute to perform.

5. Hip Circles (1 Minute): Place your hands on your hips and move them in a circle for 30 seconds in one direction and then in the opposite direction for another 30 seconds.

6. Leg lifts: Stand, lift one leg to your chest, keep it there for a moment, and then lower it. This exercise takes one minute. Legs should be switched for a minute.

7. Seated Backbend (1 minute): Put your feet flat on the floor and sit in a chair. Lean back slowly while placing your hands on your knees and slightly arching your spine. Return to an upright position after holding for a few seconds.

8. Seated Side Stretch (1 minute): To feel a stretch down your side, lift one arm above your head and bend to the other side. After a few seconds of holding, flip sides.

Advice for a Successful Warm-Up

- ❖ As you warm up, pay attention to how your body feels. Any movement that causes pain or discomfort should be changed or avoided completely.
- ❖ Stay hydrated by drinking water both before and throughout your workout.
- ❖ You are welcome to modify the warm-up exercises to fit your comfort level and any unique physical restrictions or conditions.

For seniors who do strength training, a proper warm-up regimen is crucial. It enhances performance, reduces the chance of damage, and prepares the body both physically and mentally. You may create the foundation for an excellent workout that enhances your strength, vitality, and health as you age by incorporating dynamic stretching and general warm-up exercises into your fitness regimen. Always get advice from a fitness expert or your doctor before beginning a new exercise program, particularly if you have any underlying medical conditions.

Avoiding Injuries And Identifying Signs Of Overexertion

Our overall health depends on continuing to be physically active as we age, especially through strength training. Identifying the signs of overexertion and taking preventative measures to prevent harm are as important, though. This knowledge not only increases the efficiency of exercise but also safeguards our health, enabling us to continue leading active lives for many years to come.

Overexertion occurs when the body is overworked, leading to fatigue, strained muscles, or overall damage. Elderly people need to understand their limitations and learn to listen to their bodies because their bodies might not heal as rapidly as they once did. People can prevent more serious injuries and setbacks in their fitness journey by recognizing the early signs of overexertion.

Typical Indications of Overexertion

1. Increased weariness: Although some fatigue is normal following exercise, excessive or prolonged fatigue may be a sign of overexertion. It may indicate that you overexert yourself if you experience unusual fatigue or sluggishness for a few days following an exercise session.

2. Muscle soreness and pain: New or more strenuous exercises frequently cause mild muscle soreness. On the other hand, persistent soreness that lasts for more than a few days could indicate damage or strain to the muscles. Differentiating between acute or incapacitating pain and normal discomfort is crucial.

3. Shortness of breath: Although shortness of breath might happen during intense exercise, it should rapidly return to normal after stopping. You might be overexerting yourself if you get dyspnea for longer than a few minutes or if it happens while you're sleeping.

4. Lightheadedness or dizziness: Feeling lightheaded during or after physical activity is a red flag. This can be a sign of low blood sugar, dehydration, or exertion. Stop exercising right once if you have dizziness, and if it persists, get medical help.

5. Heart palpitations: Although an elevated heart rate is normal during physical activity, if you experience irregular heartbeats or feel your heart pounding after stopping, this may be a sign of overexertion. You can stay within safe bounds when exercising by keeping an eye on your heart rate.

6. Joint pain: Although some discomfort is normal, especially when starting a new exercise program, persistent joint pain,

stiffness, or swelling could indicate an injury or overdoing it. You should pause and reevaluate your technique and exercise choices if you experience joint pain during particular motions.

7. Mood Shifts: Too much exercise can negatively impact your mental well-being by resulting in despair, frustration, or impatience. It could be time to reevaluate your fitness routine if you see significant mood changes or elevated anxiety during your workouts.

Using Wise Practices to Prevent Injuries

The first step in preventing injuries is identifying signs of overexertion. The risk of injury during strength training and other physical activities can be reduced with the use of clever strategies.

1. Start slowly and gradually: It's important for elders to gradually transition into a strength training regimen. Start with easy movements that only use your body weight or minimal resistance. As your strength and confidence grow, gradually increase the workouts' duration, intensity, and complexity.

2. Listen to your body: It's critical to develop the ability to pay attention to your body. You should quit if something doesn't

feel right. Give your body the rest it needs to recover. Don't be scared to modify or omit exercises that cause discomfort.

3. Warming up and cooling down: Adhering to appropriate warm-up and cool-down exercises can significantly reduce the risk of injury. To prepare the muscles and joints for exercise, warm up for five to ten minutes with dynamic stretches and mild cardiovascular movement. Stretch lightly when you cool down after doing exercise to improve flexibility and recovery.

4. Drink plenty of water: Dehydration can lead to fatigue, lightheadedness, and a decline in physical performance. Stay hydrated by drinking water before, during, and after workouts, particularly if the weather is hot or the exercise is demanding.

5. Select the right workouts: Select exercises that are suitable for your level of fitness and any underlying medical conditions. See a fitness expert if you're unsure if a workout program is safe and beneficial for you.

6. Maintain correct form: Keeping your form correct during exercises is crucial to preventing injuries. Avoid using momentum to finish workouts and maintain good alignment and posture. See a qualified trainer who specializes in senior fitness if you're unclear about your form.

7. Plan rest days: It's important to give your body adequate time to recuperate in between workouts to prevent overuse issues. Diversify your routines and plan frequent rest days to prevent overstressing the same muscle groups.

8. Engage in cross-training: Including a range of physical exercises will help you avoid injury and overexertion. For instance, to reduce the chance of overuse injuries and build a well-rounded fitness program, mix strength training with low-impact activities like yoga, swimming, or walking.

9. Pay attention to nutrition: Eating well supports overall health and healing. Eat a well-balanced diet rich in carbohydrates, healthy fats, and protein to support muscle recovery and fuel your workouts.

10. Speak with medical professionals: Speak with your physician or physical therapist before beginning any new exercise program, particularly if you have any underlying medical conditions. Depending on the demands and limitations of each person's health, they can provide tailored advice.

Seniors who engage in strength training must be aware of the warning signals of overexertion and know how to prevent injury. You may benefit from strength training while lowering the risks if you pay attention to your body and use safe techniques. Keep in mind that maintaining your physical health enables you to lead an active and fulfilling life, and that fitness is a lifetime endeavor. Safety should always come first, and if you have any doubts concerning your exercise regimen, don't be scared to ask for assistance.

CHAPTER 4: 60 STRENGTH TRAINING EXERCISES FOR SENIORS

Prioritizing safety and preparation is crucial before beginning your strength training regimen. For individualized guidance, people over 70 or those with pre-existing medical issues should speak with a healthcare provider. To prevent injuries and prepare the muscles and joints for activity, a complete warm-up is essential. Throughout your workouts, pay attention to your technique and pay attention to your body. If you feel pain that goes beyond typical weariness, stop and modify your routine as necessary. As you gain comfort, progressively increase the intensity of your workouts by starting with lesser weights or resistance bands.

Drink lots of water before, during, and after your workouts because staying hydrated is also crucial. Every session should conclude with a cool-down that incorporates mild stretches to promote flexibility and muscle repair. The American Council on Exercise (ACE) and the National Institute on Aging provide helpful insights on preserving health through safe exercise routines; for further advice on safe practices and exercise guidelines specific to older adults, check out their resources.

1. Spine Twist

Instructions:

1. Sit up straight on a chair with feet flat on the floor and knees bent.
2. Place your right hand on the back of the chair.
3. Twist your torso to the right, reaching your left arm across your body to hold the outside of your right knee.
4. Hold the twist for 15-30 seconds while breathing deeply, then slowly return to the center.
5. Repeat on the left side.

Benefits:

1. Enhances spinal flexibility and mobility.
2. Stimulates abdominal organs to aid digestion.
3. Relieves back and shoulder tension.

2. Chest Stretch

Instructions:

1. Sit up tall with feet flat on the ground and shoulders relaxed.
2. Interlace your fingers behind your back and straighten your arms.
3. Gently lift your arms and squeeze your shoulder blades together.

4. Hold the position for 15-20 seconds while breathing deeply.
5. Slowly release and return to the starting position.

Benefits:

1. Increases chest and shoulder flexibility.
2. Improves posture by counteracting rounded shoulders.
3. Opens the chest for improved breathing capacity.

3. Back of Thigh Stretch

Instructions:

1. Sit on the edge of a chair with your left leg extended straight in front of you.
2. Keep your back straight and slowly lean forward over your extended leg.
3. Reach toward your toes and hold the stretch for 20-30 seconds.
4. Return to the upright position and switch legs.

Benefits:

1. Increases hamstring flexibility.
2. Helps prevent lower back strain.
3. Enhances mobility for daily movements like walking.

4. Knee to Chest

Instructions:

1. Sit in a sturdy chair with your feet flat on the floor.
2. Bring one knee up toward your chest, holding it with both hands.
3. Hold the position for 15-30 seconds while keeping your back straight.
4. Lower the leg and repeat with the opposite knee.

Benefits:

1. Relieves lower back tension.
2. Improves hip flexibility and range of motion.
3. Gently stretch glutes and hamstrings.

5. Ankle Rotations

Instructions:

1. Sit comfortably and lift one foot slightly off the floor.
2. Rotate the ankle in a circular motion clockwise for 10-15 seconds.
3. Reverse the direction for another 10-15 seconds.
4. Repeat with the other ankle.

Benefits:

1. Improves ankle flexibility and range of motion.
2. Enhances blood circulation in the lower legs.
3. Helps prevent ankle stiffness and injury.

6. Seated Arm Curls

Instructions:

1. Sit up straight with feet flat on the floor and hold a light dumbbell in each hand, palms facing forward.
2. Slowly bend your elbows, bringing the weights toward your shoulders.
3. Hold briefly, then lower the weights back down in a controlled manner.
4. Perform 8-12 repetitions for each arm.

Benefits:

1. Strengthens biceps and improves arm strength.
2. Increases upper body muscle tone.
3. Enhances grip strength and coordination.

7. Bicep Curls with Resistance Band

Instructions:

1. Sit in a chair with a resistance band under your feet.
2. Hold the band with palms facing up and elbows close to your body.
3. Slowly curl the band up towards your shoulders.
4. Lower it back down in a controlled motion and repeat for 8-10 reps.

Benefits:

1. Builds bicep strength without heavy weights.
2. Improves muscle endurance in the arms.
3. Enhances joint stability in elbows and wrists.

8. Seated Row with Resistance Band

Instructions:

1. Sit on a sturdy chair with feet flat and place a resistance band under your feet.
2. Hold the band with both hands, arms extended in front of you.
3. Pull the band towards your waist, keeping elbows close to your sides.

4. Return to the starting position slowly, and repeat for 10-12 reps.

Benefits:

1. Strengthens upper back and shoulders.
2. Improves posture by targeting back muscles.
3. Increases stability in shoulder and upper arm muscles.

9. Banded Chest Press with Resistance Band

Instructions:

1. Wrap a resistance band around the back of a chair or your back.
2. Hold the ends of the band with both hands, elbows bent at your sides.
3. Press forward until arms are fully extended, then return to the starting position.
4. Perform 8-12 repetitions.

Benefits:

1. Strengthens chest, shoulders, and triceps.
2. Enhances upper body stability.
3. Improves functional movement for daily pushing activities.

10. Bent Over Row with Resistance Band

Instructions:

1. Place the middle of a resistance band under your feet and stand with feet shoulder-width apart.
2. Bend slightly at the hips and hold the band with both hands.
3. Pull the band up toward your waist, keeping elbows close to your body.
4. Lower it slowly and repeat for 10-12 reps.

Benefits:

1. Strengthens back muscles and improves posture.
2. Engages core for better stability.
3. Increases functional strength for pulling motions.

11. Chair Push-Ups

Instructions:

1. Place hands on the edge of a sturdy chair, shoulder-width apart.
2. Step your feet back to create an incline, keeping your body straight.
3. Lower your chest toward the chair, then push back up.
4. Repeat for 8-10 repetitions.

Benefits:

1. Builds chest, shoulder, and tricep strength.
2. Improves upper body endurance.
3. Boosts core stability and balance.

12. Toe Taps

Instructions:

1. Sit on the edge of a chair with feet flat on the floor.
2. Alternate lifting each foot and tapping it lightly on the floor.
3. Repeat for 15-20 taps on each foot.

Benefits:

1. Strengthens lower legs and enhances circulation.
2. Improves ankle mobility and stability.
3. Boosts coordination and foot control.

13. Extended Leg Raises

Instructions:

1. Sit tall in a chair with feet flat on the floor.
2. Extend one leg straight out, hold for a few seconds, then lower.
3. Repeat on the opposite leg, alternating for 10 reps per leg.

Benefits:

1. Strengthens quadriceps and hip flexors.
2. Increases lower body mobility and control.
3. Improves stability and posture when seated.

14. Seated Hip Marching

Instructions:

1. Sit upright with feet flat and back straight.
2. Lift one knee toward your chest, then lower.
3. Alternate legs, marching for 15-20 reps.

Benefits:

1. Improves hip mobility and leg strength.
2. Enhances coordination and balance.
3. Supports daily activities like walking and standing.

15. Calf Raises

Instructions:

1. Stand behind a chair, holding it for support.
2. Lift your heels off the ground, rising onto your toes.
3. Lower your heels slowly and repeat for 12-15 reps.

Benefits:

1. Strengthens calf muscles for stability.
2. Improves balance and lower leg endurance.
3. Enhances circulation in the lower body.

16. Ankle Circles

Instructions:

1. Sit upright in a chair and lift one foot off the floor.
2. Rotate your ankle clockwise for 10 seconds, then counterclockwise.
3. Switch feet and repeat for 10 seconds in each direction.

Benefits:

1. Enhances ankle flexibility and range of motion.
2. Improves joint mobility.
3. Reduces stiffness and enhances circulation in the ankles.

17. Chest Pull with Resistance Band

Instructions:

1. Hold a resistance band in both hands with arms extended in front of you.
2. Pull the band outward, keeping your arms straight, until you feel a squeeze in your upper back and chest.
3. Slowly bring arms back to the starting position and repeat for 10-12 reps.

Benefits:

1. Strengthens the chest, shoulders, and upper back.
2. Enhances upper body endurance and muscle tone.
3. Improves posture and stability.

18. Lateral Raise with Resistance Band

Instructions:

1. Stand with feet shoulder-width apart and step on the center of the resistance band.
2. Hold the ends of the band in each hand at your sides.
3. Lift your arms to the sides until they reach shoulder height, keeping elbows slightly bent.
4. Lower back down slowly and repeat for 10-12 reps.

Benefits:

1. Builds shoulder strength and stability.
2. Improves arm mobility and range of motion.
3. Tones and shapes shoulder muscles.

19. Band Triceps Pull with Resistance Band

Instructions:

1. Stand with one end of a resistance band under your foot.
2. Hold the other end with your opposite hand behind your head.
3. Extend your arm upward, fully straightening your elbow.
4. Lower the arm slowly and repeat for 10 reps per side.

Benefits:

1. Strengthens triceps and upper arms.
2. Improves arm extension and mobility.
3. Supports daily functional movements involving reaching and lifting.

20. Wall Push-Ups

Instructions:

1. Stand facing a wall and place your hands shoulder-width apart at chest height.
2. Step back slightly and lean toward the wall.
3. Lower your chest towards the wall by bending your elbows, then push back.
4. Perform 10-12 repetitions.

Benefits:

1. Strengthens chest, shoulders, and triceps.
2. Provides a safe, low-impact workout for upper body.
3. Helps improve posture and stability.

21. Bicep Curl with Resistance Band

Instructions:

1. Stand with your feet on the resistance band, holding the ends with palms up.
2. Keep elbows close to your body as you curl your hands toward your shoulders.
3. Lower slowly and repeat for 10-12 reps.

Benefits:

1. Builds bicep strength and endurance.
2. Increases muscle tone in upper arms.
3. Improves grip strength.

22. Partial Squats

Instructions:

1. Stand with feet hip-width apart, hands on a sturdy surface or in front of you for balance.
2. Lower yourself halfway down as if sitting, keeping your knees aligned over your toes.
3. Rise back up and repeat for 10-15 reps.

Benefits:

1. Strengthens quadriceps and glutes.
2. Increases leg endurance.
3. Supports knee stability and mobility.

23. Chair Lunges

Instructions:

1. Stand behind a chair, holding it for support.
2. Step one foot back, lowering into a lunge position.
3. Push back up, return to standing, and switch sides.
4. Repeat for 8-10 reps on each leg.

Benefits:

1. Builds leg strength and balance.
2. Increases flexibility in hips and knees.
3. Improves coordination and mobility.

24. Sit and Stand Squats

Instructions:

1. Sit on the edge of a chair with feet hip-width apart.
2. Push through your heels to stand, then slowly sit back down.
3. Perform 10-12 repetitions.

Benefits:

1. Strengthens legs, especially quadriceps and glutes.
2. Enhances functional strength for daily tasks.
3. Improves balance and stability.

25. Leg Extensions

Instructions:

1. Sit upright in a chair with feet flat on the floor.
2. Extend one leg straight out and hold for a moment.
3. Lower it back down, then switch legs.
4. Alternate for 10-12 reps on each leg.

Benefits:

1. Strengthens quadriceps and supports knee function.
2. Improves joint stability.
3. Enhances mobility in the legs for walking and standing.

26. Standing Hamstring Curl

Instructions:

1. Stand tall with your feet hip-width apart, holding onto a sturdy chair or wall for support.
2. Slowly bend one knee, bringing your heel towards your glutes. Keep your thigh straight and avoid leaning forward.
3. Lower your leg back to the starting position, and repeat on the other leg.
4. Perform 12-15 reps on each leg, focusing on engaging your hamstring throughout the movement.

Benefits:

1. Targets the hamstrings, which play a crucial role in mobility, posture, and walking.
2. Standing on one leg while performing the exercise helps enhance overall balance and stability.
3. Gently stretch the muscles at the back of your legs, improving flexibility over time.

27. Seated Leg Extension with Resistance Band

Instructions:

1. Sit on a chair with your back straight and feet flat on the floor. Secure a resistance band around your ankle and attach it to a sturdy object.
2. Slowly extend one leg out in front of you, keeping it straight, until your leg is parallel to the floor.
3. Hold for a second, then slowly lower your leg back to the starting position.
4. Repeat for 12-15 reps on each leg, keeping the movement controlled.

Benefits:

1. Targets the quadriceps, improving leg strength and endurance.
2. Helps with knee extension, which is essential for functional movements and overall knee health.
3. Enhances lower-body stability by strengthening the muscles around the knee joint.

28. Modified Burpees

Instructions:

1. Stand with your feet shoulder-width apart. Bend your knees and place your hands on the floor in front of you.
2. Step one leg back, followed by the other, into a plank position.
3. Step one leg forward, then the other, to return to the standing position.
4. Repeat for 8-12 reps, focusing on form rather than speed.

Benefits:

1. Targets the legs, core, arms, and chest, providing a full-body workout in one move.
2. Increases heart rate, improving cardiovascular health and endurance.

3. The combination of different movements challenges coordination and balance.

29. Modified Chair Plank

Instructions:

1. Sit at the edge of a sturdy chair with your hands resting on the edge. Walk your feet back so your body forms a straight line from head to heels.
2. Engage your core and hold the position for 15-30 seconds, ensuring your body remains straight.
3. Keep your shoulders directly over your wrists and avoid sagging in the hips.
4. Gradually increase the duration as your strength improves.

Benefits:

1. Engages the core muscles, promoting strength and stability.
2. Supports a healthy posture by strengthening the muscles that keep your spine aligned.
3. Strengthens the shoulders, arms, and legs, improving overall balance and stability.

30. Basic Squat

Instructions:

1. Stand with your feet shoulder-width apart and your toes pointing slightly outward.
2. Lower your hips back and down as if sitting in a chair, keeping your chest lifted and knees behind your toes.
3. Lower until your thighs are parallel to the ground, then push through your heels to return to standing.
4. Repeat for 12-15 reps, focusing on maintaining proper form throughout the movement.

Benefits:

1. Targets the quadriceps, hamstrings, and glutes, building strength in the legs and hips.
2. Enhances flexibility and range of motion in the lower body, especially in the hips and knees.
3. Helps maintain healthy knee and hip joints by promoting proper alignment and function.

31. Standing Squat Stretch

Instructions:

1. Stand with your feet wider than shoulder-width apart, toes pointing slightly outward.
2. Lower your hips back and down into a squat position, keeping your chest lifted and your knees aligned with your toes.
3. Hold the squat for 20-30 seconds, feeling the stretch in your inner thighs and hips.
4. Slowly rise to stand and repeat for 2-3 sets.

Benefits:

1. Targets the inner thighs and hips, enhancing flexibility in these areas.
2. This helps you deepen your squat while maintaining proper form.
3. Encourages the activation of lower body muscles, improving overall strength and endurance.

32. Hula Hoop Hip Stretches

Instructions:

1. Stand with your feet shoulder-width apart, holding a hula hoop (or imaginary hoop) at waist height.
2. Begin by gently swaying your hips in a circular motion, trying to mimic the movement of hula hooping.
3. Perform for 30 seconds to 1 minute in each direction, maintaining a smooth, controlled motion.
4. Repeat for 2-3 sets.

Benefits:

1. Helps stretch and loosen the hips, which can be tight from sitting or inactivity.
2. Engages the core muscles as you rotate your hips, improving overall core strength.
3. The circular motion challenges coordination and balance, enhancing overall mobility.

33. Shoulder Stretch

Instructions:

1. Stand or sit up straight with your shoulders relaxed.
2. Reach one arm across your chest, holding it with your opposite hand just above the elbow.

3. Gently pull the arm closer to your chest, feeling a stretch across your shoulder.
4. Hold the stretch for 20-30 seconds, then switch arms and repeat.

Benefits:

1. Stretches the deltoids, helping to improve shoulder mobility.
2. Releases tightness and tension in the shoulders, which is common from sitting or poor posture.
3. Enhances the range of motion in the shoulder joint, reducing the risk of injury during daily activities.

34. Chin Drop

Instructions:

1. Sit or stand with your back straight, and shoulders relaxed.
2. Slowly drop your chin toward your chest, allowing your neck to stretch.
3. Hold the position for 15-30 seconds, breathing deeply and relaxing your neck muscles.
4. Slowly return to the neutral position, and repeat 2-3 times.

Benefits:

1. Eases tightness in the neck and upper back, which can be caused by poor posture or stress.

2. By stretching the neck muscles, it can help improve overall posture.
3. Increases flexibility in the neck, reducing discomfort from prolonged sitting or computer use.

35. Arm Opener

Instructions:

1. Stand tall with your feet shoulder-width apart and arms extended in front of you at shoulder height.
2. Open your arms wide, bringing your shoulder blades together.
3. Squeeze your back muscles and hold the stretch for 15-30 seconds.
4. Bring your arms back to the starting position, and repeat for 5-10 reps.

Benefits:

1. Stretches the chest and front shoulders, helping to counteract the effects of slouching.
2. Enhances flexibility in the shoulders and upper back.
3. Promotes better posture by strengthening the muscles of the upper back.

36. Double Knee Torso Rotation

Instructions:

1. Lie on your back with your knees bent and feet flat on the floor.
2. Keep your arms out to the sides, palms facing down.
3. Slowly lower both knees to one side, keeping your shoulders on the floor.
4. Hold for a few seconds, then return to the center and rotate to the other side. Repeat for 8-12 reps per side.

Benefits:

1. Enhances rotational flexibility of the spine, improving overall mobility.
2. Gently stretches the lower back and alleviates tightness.
3. Engages the core muscles, improving balance and stability.

37. Shoulder Overhead Press

Instructions:

1. Stand with your feet shoulder-width apart, holding dumbbells or a resistance band at shoulder height.
2. Press the weights overhead, extending your arms fully.
3. Lower the weights back to shoulder height with control.

4. Repeat for 10-12 reps, focusing on maintaining a strong core and stable posture.

Benefits:

1. Targets the deltoids and other muscles of the upper body, improving shoulder strength.
2. Engages the back and core muscles to support better posture.
3. Enhances stability and muscle endurance in the shoulders and arms.

38. Shoulder Shrugs

Instructions:

1. Stand or sit with your back straight and your arms by your sides.
2. Raise both shoulders toward your ears, squeezing them at the top.
3. Lower your shoulders back down, releasing the tension.
4. Repeat for 12-15 reps, focusing on the range of motion and control.

Benefits:

1. Helps release tension from the neck and upper back muscles.
2. Targets the trapezius muscles, improving upper back strength.

3. Helps to relax tense shoulder muscles, promoting better posture and alignment.

39. Dumbbell Curl

Instructions:

1. Stand with a dumbbell in each hand, arms fully extended, and palms facing forward.
2. Curl the dumbbells toward your shoulders, keeping your elbows close to your torso.
3. Slowly lower the weights back to the starting position.
4. Repeat for 10-12 reps, focusing on controlling the movement.

Benefits:

1. Targets the biceps, improving arm strength and tone.
2. Builds muscular endurance in the arms, supporting functional movement.
3. Helps improve grip strength, which is beneficial for various daily activities.

40. One Arm Row

Instructions:

1. Stand with one foot forward, placing one hand on a bench or chair for support.
2. Hold a dumbbell in the other hand, keeping your arm extended toward the floor.
3. Pull the dumbbell towards your hip, squeezing your back muscles as you lift.
4. Lower the weight back down with control and repeat for 10-12 reps per side.

Benefits:

1. Strengthens the latissimus dorsi, rhomboids, and traps, improving posture.
2. Works the biceps and forearms in addition to the back.
3. Improves core stability by requiring balance during the exercise.

41. Seated Lateral Raise

Instructions:

1. Sit with your feet flat on the ground and a dumbbell in each hand.

2. Raise both arms to the sides until they are parallel to the ground, keeping a slight bend in your elbows.
3. Lower your arms slowly back to the starting position.
4. Repeat for 10-12 reps, ensuring controlled movement throughout the exercise.

Benefits:

1. Targets the deltoid muscles, improving shoulder strength and mobility.
2. Helps open up the chest and shoulders, counteracting slouching.
3. Builds endurance and strength in the upper body, supporting functional movements.

42. Glute Bridge Exercise

Instructions:

1. Lie on your back with your knees bent and feet flat on the floor, hip-width apart.
2. Press through your heels to lift your hips toward the ceiling, forming a straight line from your knees to your shoulders.
3. Hold the bridge position for 3-5 seconds before lowering your hips back to the floor.
4. Repeat for 10-15 reps, focusing on engaging your glutes and core.

Benefits:

1. Targets the glutes and lower back muscles, improving lower body strength.
2. Engages the core to maintain stability during the movement.
3. Strengthens the posterior chain, helping to improve posture and reduce lower back pain.

43. Bird Dog

Instructions:

1. Start in a tabletop position with your wrists under your shoulders and knees under your hips.
2. Extend your right arm forward while simultaneously extending your left leg back.
3. Hold the position for 3-5 seconds, then return to the starting position.
4. Repeat on the opposite side and continue for 10-12 reps per side.

Benefits:

1. Engages both the core and limbs, enhancing balance and coordination.
2. Targets the abdominal and lower back muscles, improving overall core strength.

3. Develops coordination between the upper and lower body, improving overall movement patterns.

44. Kneeling Shoulder Tap Push-Up

Instructions:

1. Start in a kneeling push-up position, keeping your hands under your shoulders and knees under your hips.
2. Perform a push-up by lowering your chest to the floor and pushing back up.
3. At the top of the push-up, tap your left shoulder with your right hand, then return your hand to the floor.
4. Repeat for 8-12 reps, alternating shoulder taps after each push-up.

Benefits:

1. Targets the pectorals, triceps, and shoulders.
2. Engages the core muscles to help stabilize the body during the movement.
3. The shoulder tap adds a balance challenge, promoting coordination and stability.

45. Mid Back Extension

Instructions:

1. Lie on your stomach with your arms extended in front of you and your legs straight.
2. Slowly lift your chest and upper body off the ground while keeping your lower body in contact with the floor.
3. Hold the position for a few seconds, then lower back down.
4. Repeat for 8-12 reps, focusing on using your back muscles to lift rather than your arms.

Benefits:

1. Targets the erector spinae, improving strength and stability in the lower back.
2. Helps to correct poor posture by strengthening the muscles responsible for spinal alignment.
3. Strengthening the back muscles, can reduce discomfort and the risk of back injury.

46. Sit-Ups

Instructions:

1. Lie on your back with your knees bent and feet flat on the floor, hip-width apart.

2. Place your hands behind your head or crossed over your chest.
3. Engage your core muscles and lift your upper body toward your knees, exhaling as you rise.
4. Slowly lower your upper body back to the starting position, and repeat for 10-15 reps.

Benefits:

1. Targets the abdominal muscles, improving overall core strength and stability.
2. Stronger core muscles can help improve posture and prevent slouching.
3. Increases flexibility in the spine and lower back by engaging the muscles through a full range of motion.

47. Squat Curl Knee Lift

Instructions:

1. Stand with your feet shoulder-width apart and hold a dumbbell in each hand.
2. Lower into a squat position by bending your knees and pushing your hips back.
3. As you stand back up, perform a bicep curl and lift your right knee toward your chest.
4. Repeat for 10-12 reps, alternating legs with each squat curl.

Benefits:

1. Engages the quads, hamstrings, glutes, biceps, and core muscles simultaneously.
2. Combines strength training with balance, enhancing coordination and motor skills.
3. The combination of movement patterns helps improve cardiovascular fitness.

48. Calf Raises

Instructions:

1. Stand with your feet hip-width apart and your hands resting on a chair or wall for support.
2. Slowly rise onto the balls of your feet, lifting your heels as high as possible.
3. Hold at the top for a second, then lower your heels back down.
4. Repeat for 12-15 reps, focusing on the full range of motion.

Benefits:

1. Targets the gastrocnemius and soleus muscles in the calves, enhancing lower leg strength.
2. Increases proprioception and balance by working the stabilizing muscles in the legs.

3. Encourages blood flow to the lower legs, reducing the risk of cramping and stiffness.

49. Half Squats

Instructions:

1. Stand with your feet shoulder-width apart and your arms extended in front of you for balance.
2. Bend your knees and lower your body into a squat, stopping when your thighs are parallel to the floor.
3. Push through your heels to return to the standing position.
4. Repeat for 12-15 reps, ensuring your knees don't pass over your toes.

Benefits:

1. Targets the quads, hamstrings, and glutes without putting excessive strain on the knees.
2. Helps improve flexibility and mobility in the hips, knees, and ankles.
3. Works on building strength in the legs, which supports better joint function and reduces injury risk.

50. Squat Hold

Instructions:

1. Stand with your feet shoulder-width apart and your arms extended in front of you.
2. Lower your body into a squat position, keeping your knees in line with your toes and your thighs parallel to the floor.
3. Hold the squat position for 20-30 seconds, maintaining proper form.
4. Slowly stand back up and repeat for 2-3 sets.

Benefits:

1. Targets the quads, glutes, and hamstrings, enhancing lower body strength.
2. Holds like this improve muscular endurance in the legs and core.
3. Helps strengthen the muscles responsible for maintaining good posture.

51. High Stepping

Instructions:

1. Stand with your feet hip-width apart and your arms by your sides.

2. Lift your right knee as high as possible toward your chest, then lower it back down.
3. Alternate legs, lifting each knee high in a marching fashion.
4. Repeat for 30 seconds, gradually increasing the pace.

Benefits:

1. Targets the hip flexors and thigh muscles, promoting leg strength.
2. Increases heart rate, offering a low-impact cardiovascular workout.
3. Improves joint flexibility and coordination between the upper and lower body.

52. Heel to Toe Walk

Instructions:

1. Stand with your feet together and arms at your sides.
2. Step forward with your right foot, placing your heel directly in front of your left toe.
3. Continue walking in a straight line, touching the heel of each foot to the toe of the other foot as you walk.
4. Perform this for 10-15 steps, then reverse the direction.

Benefits:

1. Helps improve balance and coordination by challenging your stability during walking.
2. Works on ankle stability and mobility, which are important for fall prevention.
3. Promotes better walking mechanics and posture.

53. Standing Hip Flexor Stretch

Instructions:

1. Stand tall and take a step back with your right foot, bending your left knee to a 90-degree angle.
2. Gently push your hips forward to stretch the front of your right hip.
3. Hold for 15-30 seconds, then switch sides.
4. Repeat 2-3 times per side for a deeper stretch.

Benefits:

1. Stretches the hip flexors, which can become tight from prolonged sitting.
2. Enhances flexibility in the hip joint, reducing stiffness.
3. Stretching the hip flexors, can help prevent back discomfort caused by tight muscles.

54. Calf Stretch

Instructions:

1. Stand facing a wall with your hands placed on it for support.
2. Step one foot back, keeping both feet flat on the ground, and bend the front knee.
3. Press your back heel into the ground, feeling the stretch in the calf.
4. Hold for 15-30 seconds, then switch legs.

Benefits:

1. Helps release tension in the calves, promoting flexibility.
2. Regular stretching can reduce the likelihood of muscle cramps.
3. Increases ankle mobility, supporting improved movement in daily activities.

55. Glute Stretch

Instructions:

1. Sit on the floor with your legs extended straight out in front of you.
2. Cross your right ankle over your left knee, forming a figure-four shape.

3. Gently press your right knee down toward the floor to deepen the stretch.
4. Hold for 20-30 seconds, then switch sides.

Benefits:

1. Helps alleviate tightness in the glutes, often caused by prolonged sitting.
2. Stretches the glute muscles, promoting better flexibility in the hips.
3. Relieving tension in the glutes can reduce lower back pain and discomfort.

56. Neck Circles

Instructions:

1. Sit or stand with your back straight and shoulders relaxed.
2. Slowly drop your chin toward your chest and rotate your head in a circular motion.
3. Perform the movement slowly in one direction for 5-10 rotations, then switch directions.
4. Repeat for 1-2 minutes, maintaining a relaxed and controlled motion.

Benefits:

1. Eases tightness and stiffness in the neck and shoulders.
2. Increases the range of motion in the neck, improving flexibility.
3. Gentle neck movements can help release stress and promote relaxation.

57. Chest Stretch

Instructions:

1. Stand with your feet shoulder-width apart and your hands clasped behind your back.
2. Straighten your arms and gently raise them to open your chest.
3. Hold the position for 20-30 seconds, breathing deeply to deepen the stretch.
4. Repeat 2-3 times for a full stretch.

Benefits:

1. Helps counteract the effects of slouching by opening up the chest.
2. By stretching the chest, it encourages better posture and alignment.
3. Releases tension in the upper back and shoulders, improving mobility.

58. Standing Quadriceps Stretch

Instructions:

1. Stand tall and hold onto a sturdy object for balance, such as a wall or chair.
2. Bend one knee and bring your foot toward your glutes, grabbing your ankle with your hand.
3. Keep your knees together and gently press your hips forward to deepen the stretch.
4. Hold the stretch for 20-30 seconds, then repeat on the other leg.

Benefits:

1. Helps lengthen the quadriceps, which are often tight from sitting or standing for long periods.
2. Increases flexibility in the front of the thighs, supporting better mobility in the hips and knees.
3. Eases tightness and discomfort in the lower body, improving range of motion.

59. Push-Ups

Instructions:

1. Start in a plank position with your hands slightly wider than shoulder-width apart and your feet together.
2. Lower your body toward the floor by bending your elbows, keeping your back straight and core engaged.
3. Push back up to the starting position, fully extending your arms.
4. Repeat for 10-15 reps, focusing on form and steady movement.

Benefits:

1. Targets the chest, shoulders, and triceps, building upper body strength.
2. Engages the core to help stabilize the body, improving overall core strength.
3. Encourages joint movement and flexibility in the wrists, shoulders, and elbows.

60. Seated Leg Extensions

Instructions:

1. Sit tall on a chair with your feet flat on the floor and your knees bent at 90 degrees.

2. Slowly extend one leg straight out in front of you, keeping
    your foot flexed and your toes pointing upward.
3. Hold the position for a few seconds, then slowly lower your
    leg back down.
4. Repeat for 10-12 reps per leg.

Benefits:

1. Targets the quads and helps improve knee joint strength.
2. Regularly performing leg extensions enhances knee
    flexibility and reduces stiffness.
3. Encourages blood flow to the lower legs, which is important
    for reducing swelling and improving circulation.

CHAPTER 5: RELAXATION AND BREATHING FOR HEALING

Breathing Techniques To Improve Relaxation And Endurance

Despite being one of the most fundamental biological processes, breathing is often taken for granted. Both mental and physical endurance can be significantly increased by comprehending and using the breath's power. This is particularly crucial for older adults since maintaining a healthy respiratory system and adopting good breathing techniques can improve general health, boost physical performance, and foster serenity. In order to improve endurance and foster calm, we shall examine various breathing strategies in this assessment.

Among the many vital functions of breathing are the removal of carbon dioxide from the body, the provision of oxygen to the body, and the regulation of biological processes. When exercising, proper breathing is essential because it guarantees that muscles get adequate oxygen to produce energy. Poor breathing, on the other hand, might result in fatigue, anxiety, and decreased performance. Learning efficient breathing techniques might help seniors with cardiovascular disease or impaired lung function increase their endurance during daily activities and exercise.

Breathing Technique Types

1. Belly breathing, or diaphragmatic respiration

The diaphragm is fully engaged during diaphragmatic breathing, which permits the lungs to expand and fill with air. This method can increase lung capacity, enhance oxygen exchange, and promote relaxation.

Instructions:

1. Choose a comfortable position to sit or lie down.
2. Two hands should be placed on your chest and abdomen, respectively.
3. Make sure your diaphragm, not your chest, rises as you take a deep breath through your nose.
4. Feel your tummy slump as you slowly release the breath through your lips.
5. Breathe for four, hold for four, and exhale for six, aiming for a moderate and consistent pattern.

By ensuring that their bodies get enough oxygen, regular diaphragmatic breathing can help seniors increase their endurance during activities.

2. Breathing with the pursed lips

A method for improving breathing during physical activity is called pursed-lip breathing. It can help elders improve their general endurance and control their breathing.

Instructions:

1. Comfortably sit or stand.
2. Take a slow, two-count breath through your nose.
3. As though you were about to whistle, purse your lips.
4. For four counts, gently and slowly exhale through pursed lips.
5. Focus on extending your exhale beyond the duration of your inhale.

By keeping airways open for longer, this method facilitates a more effective exchange of CO2 and oxygen. Elderly people who suffer from dyspnea may find it particularly helpful when exercising.

3. Square breathing, or box breathing

An organized breathing technique that promotes attention and relaxation is box breathing. It is a helpful tool for seniors who might feel uneasy or restless because it can assist reduce tension and anxiety.

Instructions:

1. Maintain a straight back when sitting comfortably.
2. Take four deep breaths through your nose.
3. For four counts, hold your breath.
4. Four times, release the breath via your mouth.
5. For four counts, hold your breath once more.
6. For many minutes, repeat the cycle.

Box breathing can help to lessen tension, promote mental clarity, and relax the mind. This method helps with relaxation and recuperation both before and after exercise.

4. Nadi Shodhana, or alternate nostril breathing.

One yoga technique that helps you relax and balance is alternate nostril breathing. For seniors seeking calm and clarity, it is the perfect exercise because it can help lower anxiety and improve focus.

Instructions:

1. Maintain a straight back when sitting comfortably.
2. Seal your right nostril with your thumb.
3. Take four deep breaths through your left nostril.
4. Using your right ring finger, close your left nostril and open your right.
5. Four times, exhale via your right nostril.

6. Take a four-count breath through your right nostril.
7. Exhale four times via the left nostril after closing the right.
8. Repeat several times.

For seniors who wish to lower stress and enhance their general well-being, this method can promote relaxation and aid in mental purification.

5. Counting breaths

A straightforward yet powerful technique for improving awareness and focus is breath counting. It can provide relaxation for elderly people who experience anxiety or restlessness.

Instructions:

1. You can easily sit or lie down.
2. Breathe deeply and close your eyes.
3. Focus on your breath and count "one" as you inhale.
4. Count "two" as you release your breath.
5. Count your breaths until you reach five, then start over at one.
6. Bring your mind back to your breathing and counting if it strays.

By bringing the attention back to the present, breath counting promotes relaxation and serenity. It works incredibly well to promote a calm mindset and stop racing thoughts.

Using Breathing Methods in Everyday Situations

These breathing techniques must be incorporated into daily routines to reap their full benefits. Seniors can benefit from the following advice:

1. Whether it's in the morning, right before bed, or right after working out, schedule time each day to practice breathing techniques.

2. Combine with Physical Activity: When walking, doing yoga, or weight training, use breathing techniques. Breathe in tandem with your movement for optimal performance and relaxation.

3. Establish a Relaxation Space: Choose a quiet, comfortable area in your home where you can do breathing exercises. This place has the potential to improve awareness and relaxation.

4. Seniors should pay attention to how their bodies react to different breathing techniques. Finding the most effective tactics and applying them consistently is crucial.

5. Seek Guidance: Elderly people who are unclear about a technique can benefit from guided sessions, which can be

conducted with the help of a healthcare professional, local workshops, or online resources.

For seniors in particular, breathing is a really helpful technique for building calm and endurance. Incorporating breathing techniques like diaphragmatic breathing, pursed-lip breathing, box breathing, alternate nostril breathing, and breath counting into everyday routines may help seniors feel more at peace and perform better physically. Adopting these habits gives people the ability to live happier, more vibrant lives in addition to improving their health.

Relaxation Methods That Support Recuperation After Exercise

Prioritizing recovery after exercise is essential for promoting body renewal and repair. For the elderly, whose bodies might need extra assistance to recuperate from physical exertion, this is especially important. Including relaxation exercises in your post-workout regimen can improve your general mood, speed up your recovery, and lessen muscle soreness. The following are some beneficial relaxation techniques for recuperation after exercise:

1. Stretching and cooling down

It's essential to cool down after working out to prevent dizziness and gradually lower your heart rate. Your cool-down activity can reduce muscle tension and increase flexibility by including a little stretching.

Instructions:

1. Static stretches for each major muscle group should be performed for 5–10 minutes after your workout.
2. During your workout, focus on the areas that were most heavily worked.
3. Stretch your arms, legs, back, and core after a strength training session.

4. For 15 to 30 seconds, hold each stretch while taking deep breaths.

Stretching eases muscle tension and soreness and increases circulation. By bringing the body from an active to a calm condition, it also promotes relaxation.

2. PMR, or progressive muscle relaxation

Each muscle group in the body can be tensed and then relaxed using the Progressive Muscle Relaxation technique. This technique can support mental calmness and help release physical stress from exercise.

Instructions:

1. Work your way up from your toes.
2. Spend five seconds tensing each muscle group, then letting go and focusing on the feeling of relaxation.
3. Take a few seconds to stretch your toes, for instance, and then relax.
4. Work your way up from your feet to your face, arms, abdomen, thighs, and calves.

PMR encourages deep relaxation and reduces tense muscles. Additionally, it can help you feel less stressed and sleep better.

3. Meditation & Mindfulness

By enabling you to remain in the moment and calm your mind, mindfulness and meditation exercises can significantly aid in your recuperation after a workout. These methods enhance overall mental and emotional well-being by encouraging self-awareness and relaxation.

Instructions:

1. Find a quiet place where you won't be bothered.
2. Maintain a straight back when sitting comfortably.
3. Shut your eyes and focus on your breathing while letting your thoughts flow freely.
4. To aid with your practice, you can also use CDs or applications that offer guided meditation.

Meditation and mindfulness can help with mental clarity, mood enhancement, and stress reduction. Frequent practice has been demonstrated to improve recovery by lowering the body's levels of the stress hormone cortisol.

4. Tai Chi or gentle yoga

After working out, doing some light yoga or tai chi will help you stretch and unwind while providing a low-impact approach to wind down. Both approaches place a strong emphasis on balance, breathing awareness, and deliberate movement.

Instructions:

1. Do a quick, mild yoga or tai chi exercise that focuses on deep breathing and quiet, controlled movements.
2. Particularly calming poses include Supine Twist, Child's Pose, and Cat-Cow Pose.

These exercises reduce muscle tension, enhance balance, and raise body awareness. They can also lessen fatigue after exercise and encourage relaxation.

5. Nutrition & Hydration

Although it's not exactly a calming method, proper nutrition and water are essential for recuperation after exercise. Eating foods high in nutrients and drinking plenty of water can help with general health and muscle recovery.

Instructions:

1. To stay hydrated, drink a lot of water after working out.
2. Think about consuming a healthy snack or meal that includes carbohydrates, protein, and good fats.
3. Whole-grain toast with avocado, a lean protein salad, or a fruit and yogurt smoothie are other options.

A healthy diet and water intake help muscles recover, reduce the risk of pain, and refill energy storage. After your workout, they also aid in general recovery, making you feel better.

6. Take a warm shower or bath

After working out, you can unwind and recuperate by having a warm bath or shower. The water's warmth promotes circulation and relaxes aching muscles.

Instructions:

1. Unwind for 15 to 20 minutes in a warm bath or shower after working out.
2. Use Epsom salts or fragrant oils like lavender to help you relax even more.

Warm water eases fatigue and soothes tense muscles. You can relax after working out because of the tranquil surroundings, which also encourage mental relaxation.

7. Mild Motion

After an exercise session, light movement can improve blood circulation and reduce stiffness, which will aid in the healing process. Walking and mild cycling are examples of light exercises that can keep the body moving without overtaxing the muscles.

1. After your main workout, think about stretching lightly or taking a ten to fifteen-minute walk.
2. To enjoy the advantages of nature and fresh air, this can be done outdoors.

Mild movement eases stiffness and soreness by removing metabolic waste products from the muscles. It can also improve mood and well-being.

For seniors in particular, incorporating relaxation techniques into your post-workout regimen is essential for optimal recuperation. Improved healing and overall well-being are facilitated by stretching, deep breathing, progressive muscle relaxation, mindfulness, gentle yoga, and drinking enough water. Seniors who prioritize these activities can encourage a healthier and more active lifestyle by developing a sense of calm and relaxation in addition to aiding in their physical recovery.

CHAPTER 6: ESTABLISHING ATTAINABLE, INSPIRING OBJECTIVES AND MONITORING RESULTS

Any effective strength training program must include setting attainable, inspiring goals and effectively monitoring progress, especially for seniors over 70. It is impossible to overstate the importance of having a well-defined objective and a trustworthy tracking system as people set out on their fitness journeys. In addition to promoting dedication, this approach enables seniors to monitor their development, which improves their health and general well-being.

The Significance of Goals

Goals act as a roadmap, guiding people to the results they want. Seniors may become more motivated and focused if they set SMART goals—specific, measurable, achievable, relevant, and time-bound. Seniors can stay on track by setting clear goals, whether they are to improve general fitness, balance, or muscle strength.

Goal Types

1. Short-term Objectives: These can be accomplished in a few weeks or months and act as stepping stones to more ambitious objectives. A short-term goal can be to stretch frequently to increase flexibility or to perform a specific number of exercises three times a week.

2. Long-term Objectives: These are overarching objectives that may require months or even years to accomplish. Examples include maintaining independence in day-to-day tasks, lifting a certain weight, and completing a certain number of repetitions of an exercise.

Setting SMART objectives

Goals should adhere to the SMART criteria to be effective:

1. Specific: Clearly define your objectives. Instead of saying, "I want to get stronger," include, "I want to do 10 consecutive wall push-ups."

2. Measurable: Provide criteria for gauging advancement. For instance, "I want to increase my dumbbell curl weight from 5 lbs to 10 lbs in three months."

3. Achievable: Establish realistic objectives based on your current level of physical fitness. For instance, "I will practice seated leg raises three times per week."

4. Relevant: Verify that the goal aligns with your driving forces and general health goals. A target that would be pertinent if balance improvement is important would be "I want to hold a single-leg balance for 10 seconds."

5. Time-bound: Set a deadline for finishing the task. Like this: "Within four weeks, I want to increase my calf raises to 15 repetitions."

Techniques for Maintaining Motivation

1. Discovering Your Motivation

Seniors could tie their objectives to their own passions or dreams to increase motivation. Aligning objectives with these interests increases commitment, whether it's playing with grandchildren, attending social gatherings, or just having more freedom.

2. Including Pleasure

The procedure is more fulfilling when enjoyable hobbies are chosen. Enjoyment is crucial for maintaining motivation, whether it means selecting engaging activities or altering routines to prevent boredom. For instance, taking a group class can help you reach your fitness objectives and promote social interaction.

3. Encouragement

Maintaining motivation requires acknowledging and applauding small victories. Recognizing achievements fosters a feeling of satisfaction, whether it's reaching a goal or completing a challenging workout. This could be treating oneself to a favorite pastime or gathering with loved ones to celebrate achievements.

4. Systems of Support

Strength training with loved ones, friends, or neighborhood organizations helps keep you motivated and accountable. Attending a local fitness class or working out with a partner offers a support system that encourages regularity and a feeling of community.

5. Monitoring Development

Monitoring one's progress is essential for assessing one's success and spotting areas for development. This feedback loop makes it possible to adjust goals as necessary and boosts motivation.

Ways to Monitor Development

1. Fitness Journals: Using a notebook to document workouts, exercises, sets, repetitions, and weight changes might be beneficial. This approach produces a transparent record of development and can help spot trends over time.

2. Technology and applications: Wearable technology and fitness apps can be used to track heart rates, log workouts, and determine overall activity levels. To make tracking more engaging, a lot of apps let users set goals, log exercises, and see progress graphs.

3. Progress photos: Especially when it comes to strength, muscular tone, and general fitness, taking pictures at regular intervals can help show progress. Due to the ability to visually assess their progress over time, seniors may find this technique motivating.

4. Frequent Evaluations: Determining strength and endurance gains can be facilitated by setting up predetermined timeframes for tracking progress, such as once a month or every few weeks. This may entail figuring out the maximum weight to lift, the maximum number of repetitions, or the amount of flexibility to increase.

5. Fitness Tests: Timed sit-to-stand tests and other basic fitness tests can help detect changes in functional mobility and

strength. There are clear indicators of success when these tests are reviewed on a regular basis.

A good strength training program for adults over 70 must include setting attainable, inspiring goals and monitoring progress. Setting SMART goals, developing self-motivation, utilizing a variety of tracking methods, and maintaining flexibility when modifying objectives can all help seniors create a fulfilling fitness journey that enhances their strength, mobility, and overall quality of life. By deciding to embrace a better and more active lifestyle and sticking with it, they can achieve amazing results.

CONCLUSION

Congratulations on taking the first step towards becoming a stronger, healthier, and more independent version of yourself. This masterwork is more than simply a workout guide; it's a road plan for regaining your vigor and confidence at any stage of life.

You've already learned that strength exercise, when done right and safely, can be life-changing. Whether you're just getting started with fitness or want to push yourself farther, the workouts in this book are designed to be simple, effective, and adaptable. Remember that growth is individualized, and there is no one-size-fits-all solution. Your path is about developing strength at your speed, with no rush.

Throughout the chapters, you've learned about a range of exercises designed specifically for seniors to increase mobility, strength, bone health, and balance. Aside from the physical benefits, strength training improves your emotional and mental well-being. Lifting weights, doing bodyweight exercises, and committing to a fitness routine, as demonstrated in many of the accounts in this book, can provide a great sense of accomplishment and empowerment.

As you continue your training, remember to cherish the tiny victories. These successes are important, whether they involve standing a bit taller, climbing stairs more easily, or feeling more enthusiastic throughout the day. Strengthening takes time, but every exercise, stretch, and deep breath you take brings you closer to the vibrant, independent life you deserve.

Those who have read this book and found strength should realize that their journey is only just beginning. Maintain consistency, patience, and commitment to your health. For those just getting started, believe that with time, you will notice the tremendous changes that occur from focusing on your physical well-being. You, like the many seniors who have already embraced this book, will get life-changing benefits from strength training.

Strength is more than simply muscle. It's all about confidence. It's all about freedom. It's about understanding you can take charge of your health and future.

So let us continue our trip together. Your stronger self awaits you, and with this book, you will be well prepared to meet it.

Here's to a healthier, more independent you today and in the years to come.